Pregnancy Guide:

Step-By-Step Guide For First Time Mommies

Table of content

Introduction

First I would like to congratulate you on becoming a new mommie-to-be and for downloading this book **"Pregnancy Symptoms, Special Diet and Exercises and Week-to-Week Guide Through Your Pregnancy."** To make the book easier for you to follow I have classified the book into the three trimesters each with month-to-month descriptions and explanations of what you can expect and what happens throughout the different stages of your pregnancy. Even if you have not yet conceived, but are planning to or if you are already a month or two pregnant, I am sure you will still find the information in this book helpful and useful to you.

You are going to go through a lot of different changes both emotionally and physically during your 40 week pregnancy. Reading this book is going to help you prepare both psychologically and physically for giving birth. Of course you will also have the support of your loved ones around you doing this time. It is important that after conception that you have good healthcare and taking care of your emotional well-being to help make your pregnancy go as smoothly as possible. Finding a suitable form of exercise for yourself is going to help keep you in top physical shape during your pregnancy, this can really do wonders for you going through the different stages of pregnancy. Of coarse making sure that you are giving yourself a good nutritional diet during this time will help to ensure that you and your baby will stay in good health. Try to help and understand yourself during this time and do as much as you can for yourself as possible.

Even if you are not pregnant at this time, but you are planning to become pregnant it is a good idea to make sure that you understand what you will be experiencing during those 40 weeks of being pregnant. It is important that you are aware what you need to do to ensure that you will be doing the right things to protect your health and that of your unborn child. When you have read this book it will make you more aware of what things you need to do to prepare for your pregnancy and what you can expect during the different trimesters of your pregnancy. You will feel more comfortable and confident if you have done your research and know what will be involved during those 40 weeks of pregnancy. You are going to be more able to cope if you know what to expect and how you should handle different situations that may arise during your pregnancy.

Chapter 1 – Your First Trimester

It may surprise you to learn this, but your pregnancy occurs two weeks before you conceive. Before you conceive, you undergo what is called ovulation. During this time you release a mature egg from your ovary and it is then pushed to the fallopian tube in preparation for becoming fertilized. During this time, the lining of the uterus thickens in preparation for the fertilized egg but if the egg does not become fertilized, the wall of the uterus will shed off and this is what is known as menstruation. When your egg leaves your ovary it lives for about 24 hours in the fallopian tube. Sperms can live up to 72 hours which means the chances of pregnancy a day or two during and after the ovulation period are very high. If your egg becomes fertilized, it implantation takes about six to twelve days after ovulation. At this point the sex of the baby is determined, blending the father's and mother's traits from the ovum and the sperm cell combination. However you cannot really tell whether it is a boy or girl because at inception, the genitals look alike whether it is a boy or girl. All fertilized eggs usually have a little bud or tiny swelling or genital hub. Testosterone starts to be produced at seven weeks, if you are having a boy. At this point the buds grow and develop into a penis and scrotum for a boy and a labia and clitoris for a girl. This is a very gradual process so don't be too anxious in the first trimester to go for tests. You will more than likely not know that you are pregnant on the day the egg becomes fertilized.

Third Week
The process of fusion of the sperm and egg continues. The newly created life begins the process of cell division, which it needs to do so that the growth process can resume. The baby at this time has already began to develop the features of a human being, they are not visible at this point to the human eye.

Fourth Week

Your baby will be weighing about three ounces by the end of the fourth week and will be about one centimeter long. It is a very overwhelming time when you find out that you are pregnant it may be a joyous moment or cause some fear if you were not prepared for this pregnancy to occur. You will know that you are pregnant when you miss a few periods or menstrual cycles. This is especially true if you are someone that has regular cycles. It is best to go and have a pregnancy test to confirm everything. Your doctor will test the presence of HCG (Human chorionic gonadotropin) hormone in the urine. Another way is to test your blood 7-12 days after conception. Your uterine will start to enlarge around 8 weeks into your pregnancy. This is also another way of detecting whether you are pregnant. In the early weeks of pregnancy to find out for sure if you are pregnant you will need to visit your doctor to be examined. Around twelve weeks into your pregnancy a Doppler can be used to detect your child's heart beat.

An ultrasound will be able to determine when your delivery date will be seven weeks into your pregnancy.

Good diet

During this important time in your life it is very important that you make sure to plan a good diet for yourself during your pregnancy. You should try to be active as much as possible and eat a variety of healthy foods and get plenty of rest. This will help ensure the good health of you and your child. Not only will you be relying on your body to provide good healthy energy sources, but so will your unborn child. Within the first month of pregnancy your uterus will begin to slowly transform. During this time you will likely experience some per-menstrual cramping. During this time there is also an increase in your metabolic rate, this will cause an increase in the frequency of urination. You may also feel faint and exhausted for short periods of time. You will also feel that your breasts are getting tender during this time because your mammary glands are triggered into start maturing.

You Could Experience

You are going to experience different physical, behavioral, and hormonal changes in your first month of pregnancy. Knowing what to expect will help you prepare psychologically for when they do happen. Common pregnancy symptoms you will experience are:

∞ Morning sickness this gives you a feeling of nausea accompanied with vomiting. These are major signs of early pregnancy. Not all women experience these symptoms. Some women may feel a slight discomfort with their stomach while others may become slightly ill. Some women may go through a period where they are vomiting at least once a day. If you are going through this you should not worry too much as it will eventually go away. It is not sure what causes this, but some believe it is a result of the sudden hormonal changes or imbalances in early pregnancy.

∞ Softening of the cervix is one sign that medics use to determine pregnancy.

∞ Increased body temperatures after ovulation, your temperature levels will increase. This will stay with you for the first few weeks after you have conceived.

∞ Frequent urination three weeks after conception due to the increased pressure on the bladder, due to the increase of metabolism, this increases urination. This should decrease after the second trimester of your pregnancy, it will return near the end of your pregnancy as the pressure from your growing uterus shifts into the pelvis affecting your bladder.

∞ During your pregnancy you will not have a period. There should be no menstrual flow at this time. This is due to the embryo is now implanted on the wall or lining that is supposed to shed off when fertilization does not take place. If it happens that your period is late you might want to consider that you may be pregnant. Becoming aware of the early symptoms of pregnancy you will have a better more clear idea if you are pregnant.

Taking Care of Yourself During the First Month of Your Pregnancy

From the early stages of your pregnancy you must begin to make sure that you are eating properly. To help with the development of your baby you need to be on a good diet plan. To make sure that you do not gain too much weight during pregnancy keep doing exercises. At this point in your pregnancy you do not need to eat for two people. Making sure to do regular exercise will help get you back to your regular weight much easier after your pregnancy. But you need to expect to gain weight during your pregnancy. You should make sure to set up some savings to cover the cost for delivery and other associated cost with pregnancy.

Second Month

During the second month of your pregnancy your baby will continue to develop it's major organs such as the brain and spinal column. Your baby's heart will begin to beat by the 5th week. Internal organs continue to develop during this time. By the time the sixth week roles around in your pregnancy your baby is going to measure one quarter of an inch from head to toe. Your baby's arms and legs begin to form, as well as the mouth. By the seventh week your baby's arms and legs begin to lengthen, you will be able to tell the difference between the shoulder and forearm. You cannot see fingers at this point of the pregnancy. Eyes and nostrils continue to develop further at this point.

The eyes will look large and open always at this stage. The umbilical cord will continue to lengthen and the heart of your baby is visible as it is bulging out.

During the eighth week your baby will continue to develop its organ systems and by the eighth week your baby will have all the necessary features of a normal human being. At this point its bones will begin to harden. All these amazing changes will be occurring inside your womb. You too will experience changes in your own body in different ways. It is common to have mood swings in the second month. It is not uncommon to experience mood fluctuations.

Third Month

In the third month the facial features of your baby will begin to show, the outer ears, and nostrils are clearly distinguishable. You will be able to feel movements of your baby so don't get too freaked out when your baby begins to move its head around. Your fetus is now three inches long at this stage, with all of its internal organs developing. By the end of your third month that is when your hormones should become stabilized leaving you with less of the "moody" feelings. You will become less likely to be throwing tantrums. Now this does not mean that you will certainly experience these mood swings during pregnancy, but a great deal of women when pregnant do experience them. It certainly will not hurt for you to be psychologically prepared for them. By the third month the risk of miscarriage decreases. This being said you should still take care to make sure that you are eating the proper foods that lean towards a healthy lifestyle because a miscarriage cannot be completely ruled out. Lifestyle changes you may want to consider while pregnant.

Caffeine

Too much caffeine is not only bad for you but also not good for your baby. Any woman at the child bearing age should not take more than 300 mgs of caffeine daily. In this total are included natural sources as well such as herbs like the yerba mate and Guarana. Make sure to limit the amount of tea and coffee that you are consuming during pregnancy. You would be better to lean more towards healthier alternatives such as water, pure fruit juice, and milk. These healthy drinks will provide your baby with essential nutrients. You should stay away from tea while you are pregnant. Especially teas such as chamomile and other herbal teas are not good for you while pregnant. Teas that are considered safe during pregnancy are linden flower and citrus peel.

Changes During the First Trimester of Pregnancy and How to Deal with Them
To begin with it is a good practice not to skip meals whether you are pregnant or not. When you are pregnant you do not have the luxury to skip meals. You need to ensure that you are eating a healthy and balanced diet throughout your pregnancy. The proteins of your body are the building blocks working in collaboration with other important nutrients. Your baby needs these important nutrients in order to remain healthy and grow. You will help your baby to build tissues, body organs, and bones by providing it with good quality proteins.

Take more carbohydrates in the first three months to give you more energy and energize your baby for more healthy growth. Most women find that their appetite is reduced in the first three months of pregnancy. Often they feel too tired and sick to eat.

To help deal with this problem eat healthy food choices as they will help reduce much of these symptoms. In the first trimester you are going to need more calcium and vitamin D, especially during the second month to help aide in the growth of teeth and bones for your baby. Vitamin D is good in helping absorb calcium and using it. Eating enough calcium will also help your own bones and teeth stay healthy.

Start to consume more foods that are rich in calcium, such as milk. You can also get calcium from foods such as yogurt and cheese. You might want to come up with a diet plan that will work for you especially if you are nausea. In the second and third months of pregnancy you are probably going to have some food cravings. Women during pregnancy often experience food cravings during the third month of pregnancy. You can have some of the foods that you are cravings as long as you are getting the nutrients that you and your baby need.

You may find that you are craving weird non-food things such as clay or dirt. If this is happening it could be that you are lacking in iron. Your body is responding by looking for ways to get some iron. It could also be a sign that you are anemic or developing anemia. You should visit your doctor to get advice on what to do.

Planning Meals for Yourself

It is important that you make a well-balanced meal plan for yourself especially when you know you are pregnant. Your developing baby needs all the nutrients to develop and grow normally so you must eat healthy. You can prevent chances of anemia, by eating healthy. It can also reduce your chances of miscarriage, and reduced immunity or giving birth to a pre-mature baby or one with a low birth weight. Even though it is good that you eat more food it does not mean to go on an eating spree. Adding an extra 300 calories to your daily diet will be just fine. Health foods are high in proteins, and low in fats, and low in sugars. Most pregnant women intake about 1800 calories in the first trimester. You can start to manage your weight early in the pregnancy.

Dealing with Your Emotions During Pregnancy

During the first three months of pregnancy you will find that your emotions will shift from happy, anxiety to sadness. You could get weighed down with stress now and again. You need to learn to cope with these shifts in moods and feelings. Don't worry too much about gaining weight, don't let this get you down. Instead just make sure to take the recommended amount of calories. If your realize that you are gaining weight just remember that this is a normal part of being pregnant. You can work at shedding off the excess weight after your pregnancy.

At this point your main focus should be to make sure that your baby is safe/ healthy throughout the pregnancy. Don't worry about your weight unless it is getting to a point where it is threatening your health and your babies. Eating the right foods will also improve your emotions.

You need to keep your emotional health in constant check. If your emotions are getting too out of hand for you then seek the help of a counselor. So you should be prepared to expect heightened mood changes during your first trimester of pregnancy. But it shouldn't be too much that you cannot handle.

Prenatal Visits

A good time to have your prenatal visit is at the end of your third month of pregnancy. Seek help from a healthcare provider in your area they will be able to offer you assistance in dealing with any worries or concerns that may arise during your pregnancy.

Exercise

During the first trimester in the third month you will notice weight gain as your body will be growing to accommodate the growing baby. Do not spend too much time worrying about your weight during pregnancy. It is best for you and your baby that you continue to do regular exercise throughout your pregnancy. It will help you feel more comfortable and have more energy during your pregnancy. You can do things such as go swimming or take a walk. You could also do some shopping to keep yourself busy instead of laying around the house all day. But you should not over do it either and take some rest when you feel that you need it. Your body is going to be pretty busy 24/7 with the development of your baby. So when you are feeling tired get some rest. Find a position where you can feel comfortable and get rid of the stress and stay calm. You can exercise for 30 minutes a day.

In the first trimester, the exercises that are recommended are those that focus on stamina, muscle, and core strength. These kind of exercises will help to strengthen your waist, abdomen, back and pelvis giving your body the strength it will need to support your weight gain during pregnancy. This will mainly be in the belly area. Do some warm ups that will help prepare you for your workout.

During your second trimester you can try to do cardio workouts such as walking one a treadmill on a slow speed or you can take a nice walk making sure to keep yourself hydrated by drinking lots of water.

Times not to exercise

Although exercise is recommended during pregnancy, there is some circumstances when it should not be done. The reason being as it could end up doing more harm than good. If you suffer from certain disease you should refrain from exercises. Such diseases as the following:

Chronic bronchitis, heart disease, or severe asthma, migraines, dizziness, chest pain, calf pain or swelling, muscle weakness, vaginal bleeding, or fluid leaking, shortness of breath, risk of preterm labor. It is best to consult with your doctor to see if they think you can do exercise during your pregnancy or not.

During your pregnancy you will have to cut back on the intensity and length of your workouts.

Exhaustion

Many pregnant women complain of fatigue during their first trimester. This is due to the fact that you have a growing baby inside of you that is using your body's resources. Your own body is secreting more progesterone—this is the hormone that is known for its sedating effect. So it makes sense that you would feel tired. You can take care of yourself during this time by:

∞ slowing down with some things and cutting back on others

∞ don't overdue things such as doing housework

∞ take a nap when you feel tired and make sure to go to bed early

∞ cut back on the intensity of your workouts

∞   doing exercise is going to help you build your strength

Queasiness

Your body increases the production of Estrogen during early pregnancy. Estrogen tends to trigger nausea and vomiting in many women during early pregnancy. To help you to stop feeling less queasy during the day you should:

∞   eat smaller meals more frequently

∞   stay away from spicy foods

∞   keep saltine crackers (many women find them helpful)

∞   have ginger tea or juice to help soothe your stomach

Frequent Urination

Your uterus continues to expand and grow as it does it will put more pressure on your bladder and you will find yourself peeing frequently. Take this in stride as this just means that your baby is growing. It can get very tiring when you have to go every few minutes. To help with this situation you should:

∞   stop taking caffeine at night as it will only stimulate your bladder

∞   stop drinking liquids a few hours before you go to bed

∞   drink lots of liquids throughout your day

Tender Breasts

When you are pregnant this is accompanied with breast milk production. Before this can happen your body must prepare for this. You may experience tender swollen breasts or even sore nipples due to the surge of hormones as your body prepares your breasts for their milk producing function. It is important that you:

∞ find a comfortable bra—one that is made from soft stretchy material, no underwires

∞ wear a tank top when you go to sleep at night

∞ or you can wear a soft cotton sleep bra

Dry Eyes

Your blood circulation will become increased during pregnancy. Even though this is good it will cause your body to feel swollen. Your eyes will be affected by this causing the corneas to curve and thicken. You will notice a change in your vision. You may have to stop wearing contacts and use only glasses. On the other hand if your eyes are good you may still suffer from dry eyes. Use eye drops to keep your eyes lubricated.

Acne

You may have heard that your skin becomes nice and soft during pregnancy. Well the opposite could also happen due to the hormonal production. When your hormones work overtime it causes your skin to break out and produce more oil. You should:

∞ wash your skin very gently instead of scrubbing it

∞ use and oil-free moisturizer

∞ avoid products that contain salicylic acids, benzoyl peroxide, and steroids as these are bad for your baby.

Headaches

Headaches can be very common during pregnancy. Your metabolism changes during this time which can lead to low blood sugar. You should:

∞ massage your temples

∞ get plenty of fresh air

∞ use cold or hot compress

∞ consult your doctor if you are suffering from migraines

Changes that you shouldn't ignore

Aside from the usual changes you will undergo during pregnancy there may be some that will require medical attention. These are:

∞ heavy bleeding during your pregnancy

∞ you may experience light spotting during your pregnancy

∞ don't be alarmed it is usually not a problem when it is just light spotting

∞ if you are having heavy bleeding you should see your doctor

∞ feeling queasy or sick throughout the day is normal, but if it gets to a point where you are unable to eat anything you need to see your doctor

∞ you need to get this sorted so that you do not suffer from electrolyte imbalance and dehydration.

∞ Also talk to your doctor if six hours pass and you have not had a pee.

∞ If you are having constant belly aches go see your doctor.

∞ You will feel an odd twinge here and there in your lower abdomen during the first trimester, but if it turns into a steady pain, seek medical advice. This kind of pain could be signaling an ectopic pregnancy.

∞ If you are suffering from frequent constipation you should seek medical advice.   It is not unusual to experience some constipation during pregnancy. But you should not be going past three days without a bowel movement. If this happens you need to talk to your doctor.

Chapter 2 – Second Trimester

The second trimester of your pregnancy covers the fourth, fifth and sixth months of your pregnancy. At this stage of your pregnancy this is a bit more relaxed compared to the first trimester. There are no major changes during this time except the expected ones like the growth of your child and your tummy increasing in size to accommodate your growing baby. There are other biological and physical changes that happen too. Let us take a closer look into what you can expect in the second trimester of your pregnancy.

Fourth Month

By the time you roll into the fourth month of your pregnancy you can expect your baby's heart beat to be stronger than before. The fine hair of the baby develops and the fetus at this point is around six inches long weighing about four ounces.

Tip: You may experience heightened constipation during your fourth month of pregnancy. The reason being is that food is passing very slowly so that you and your baby are able to get extra nutrients from the foods.

Fifth Month

During the fifth month of pregnancy your baby's toes and fingernails will have formed. At this time your baby will begin to react to noise. Therefore try to avoid things that will send shocks to your baby such as a very noisy environment. You are also going to feel that your baby's movements are much more vigorous than before. The fetus will be twelve inches long and one pound at this point in the pregnancy.

Sixth Month

Your babies eyes are now open. Amniotic fluid which is a creamy substance will cover your baby during this period; this will help keep your baby hydrated, and also helps to absorb shock. The baby's skin usually looks wrinkled at this point, and the baby looks thin at about 14 inches long and weighing about one and half pounds.

Ways for You to Deal with Change in the Second Trimester
Nutrition

To avoid the problem of constipation make sure to eat foods that are high in fiber. During this duration eating lots of fruits and vegetables will be very important for you. Also try to consume more whole grains, cooked beans, lentils, and peas. Drink lots of fluids more often especially warm water to help hydrate your body and enhance digestion.

Do not use laxatives to treat constipation when you are pregnant. These could end up causing contractions that could lead to a miscarriage. Before using any type of medications you should seek the advice of your doctor first.

During the fifth month of pregnancy it is highly advised to use iron supplements. It is important for you to have enough healthy blood, iron is necessary for you as an expectant mother. Your baby also needs this iron to help build up its blood tissues to be used after birth. If your baby is lacking in iron it could cause illness to it after delivery. It could even cause slow learning and mental retardation.

Make sure to take in foods that are rich in iron as often as possible. Foods such as red meat, whole grains, eggs, poultry, canned beans, lentils, cereals, and enriched breads are all very good sources of iron. Make sure to practice moderation if you are already taking an iron supplement. Do not overdo it as we know that too much of anything is not always good.

During the second trimester of your pregnancy you should be eating 2200 calories a day at least. Cereals, bread, pasta, and rice at this point are good for your health.

Eat about ten servings a day of carbohydrates so that you and your baby will get the energy that you both need for growth. With whole-grain foods you will get folic acid and iron. You can get iron, magnesium, vitamin A from veggies. Eat for or five servings of veggies a day and four to five servings of fruit a day. Fruits will provide you with vitamin A, C and fibers, as well as potassium. Eat as much fresh fruit and fresh juice as you can. Have three servings a day of dairy products such as milk, yogurt and cheese. These will be good sources of phosphorous, protein and calcium. They also offer vitamin B, iron and zinc. You also need fat in your diet. Your growing baby will need fat for energy and for the development of its brain. You need to contact your doctor if you have a special diet to make sure that you are eating right.

During the sixth month of your pregnancy you will need to continue working on your nutrition. Drinking lots of milk, eating yogurt. Increasing your fruit and veggie intake. Eat foods such as carrots, squash, cabbage, rolled oats, apples, meat, fish, lentils, and poultry.

Gestation Diabetes
Near the end of your second trimester it would be a good idea to be tested for Gestation diabetes. Due to the abnormally high levels of sugar during pregnancy it can result in gestation diabetes. This is a common health problem with many pregnant women. Keep a close eye on your sugar levels during pregnancy. According to your BMI (body mass index) eat a well-planned diet. Talk to a dietitian they can help you to come up with a suitable meal plan for you during your pregnancy. To keep your glucose levels stabilized your diet should be made up of a good balance of fats, proteins, and carbohydrates.

Exercising

You need to keep being physically active while you are pregnant. Most women tend to become more relaxed and less active in their second trimester. Moving little is not good for your health. You need to walk around regularly to ensure that your muscles are functioning at their best.

During your second trimester you should focus on exercises that will help stabilize your posture, core and balance. Doing these kinds of exercises will aide your spine in maintaining an upright position, these will help protect your back as your belly continues to protrude further. A nice light exercise can help you to maintain your balance as well. Engaging in using your deep core muscles, spine muscles, and hips will be very beneficial to you. These kind of exercises will also help your body to recover quickly after the delivery of your baby.

You can do a warm up for your workout of five or ten minutes of stretches, doing shoulder rolls and knee lifts.

Note: Make sure to take a rest in between every set of exercise or take a rest when you feel that you need to, don't over exert yourself during this time.

Exercise Suggestions

Tummy Sucking. Pretend that you are inhaling your stomach and exhale by relaxing your abdominal muscles to help pull your belly toward your belly button. Do this exercise repeatedly.

Sitting Cycling. You can do sitting cycling at least 20 times for each leg in a day.

Kegel Exercises. Sit on a chair or even on a bed and squeeze your pelvic floor muscle by contracting inwards tightly and holding for a few seconds. If you are unsure how to do this just imagine you are peeing then stop in mid pee and hold and release, doing this repeatedly.

Squats with a Chair. Using a chair hold onto it and make sure not to lose your balance. Spread your legs apart and lower yourself by bending your knees, sticking your bottom out, and lean forward at the waist.

Hair Growth

You may find you will experience hair growth, this is great, as long as it is growing where you want it to. During pregnancy hormones tend to cause a boost in hair growth, on your back, face, and arms. You may want to get rid of this excess hair by using techniques such as laser removal, or waxing, or electrolysis but don't do this; instead use tweezers or shaving. It may be difficult for you to tweeze or shave, but these are the safer bet during pregnancy.

Congestion & Nosebleeds

Hormonal changes during pregnancy can be responsible for causing your mucus membranes to swell. You may find yourself with a stuffy nose and even snoring at night. You may also find yourself experiencing nose bleeds. Use saline drops, check with a healthcare provider if you want to use decongestant. Try using a humidifier as this will help keep the air moist. If your nose bleeds keep your head straight and pinch your nostrils, do not tilt head back this will just add to congestion.

Body shape Changing

During the second trimester is when your body is making visible changes. Your hips will widen and your belly will be growing. You are going to have to invest in some maternity clothes. You should be able to find clothes that will fit your pregnancy type. You can get clothes that will be comfortable but stylish. You want to choose styles that are easy to get in and out of especially when you will be going to the bathroom for pee breaks a lot more often. You may also experience stretch marks with your changing body. Usually these marks will fade away after childbirth so no need to worry.

Sex Drive

During your second trimester your sex drive will change due to the overdrive production of estrogen. For many pregnant women their morning sickness is replaced with sexual arousal feelings. However some women do not want to engage in sex because they have hypersensitivity caused by more blood flow to the vagina. Talk to your partner to decide how to proceed with your situation.

Vaginal Discharge

It is very common to have vaginal discharge during pregnancy. A milky white discharge is nothing to worry about it could make you uncomfortable. Use a pantyliner to catch discharge. If you notice that the discharge is yellow or green and has a foul smell this could mean an infection. Your doctor can prescribe the needed drugs to combat the infection you may experience.

Bleeding Gums

The increase of blood flow when you are pregnant can increase the blood flow to your gums due to hormonal changes. This can lead to you having swollen gums. Your gums can become more sensitive and bleed easily. Gently floss and get a softer toothbrush. Do not skip dental hygiene as gum disease increases when you are pregnant.

Changes You Shouldn't Ignore

There are certain changes that should give a red flag signal to you. When you experience these types of changes you need to contact your doctor. Symptoms for concern are:

∞ severe dizziness

∞ rapid weight gain

∞ severe abdominal pain

∞ bleeding

Chapter 3 – Third Trimester

The third trimester is the last trimester of your pregnancy that covers the seventh, eighth and ninth month.

Seventh Month

Your fetus weighs at this point in the pregnancy about 2.5 pounds and it is around 15 inches in length. Most women will have swollen feet and ankles at this point in their pregnancy. The swollen feet and ankles is called edema. Don't worry if you experience this; it is simply because when you are pregnant you will be retaining more water in your body. So at this point you should try and cut down on your fluid intake. It does not mean that you should go without water and other essential fluids by any means. You still need to drink more milk for your good health.

Eighth Month

By the time you are in the eighth month of your pregnancy your fetus will weigh around five pounds and be about 18 inches in length. You are going to feel heavy around this time. You will most likely get heartburn often during your third trimester. The pressure that is caused by your growing baby and hormonal changes can cause your food in your stomach to up your throat quite often. Stomach acid also moves up, causing the burning sensation in your chest.

Ninth Month

Your baby will weigh about eight pounds at this point and be about 20 inches in length. Your baby's skin will be less wrinkled and it's eyes will be opening and shutting. The fetus at this point will be able to react to light. During the ninth month it will be important that you drink lots of water and other essential fluids because your baby will be thirsty most likely during this point of pregnancy. Water will help transfer nutrients from your body to your baby's body. Water also carries away your waste products and your baby's waste products. Water will also help you to keep your body cool this will lessen your chances of constipation. Keep in mind that more than half of your body weight is made up of water so keep drinking fluids. The hormone that triggers milk production will be released from your placenta and your breasts will get fuller. They will not be too pronounced until your baby is born. Around the end of the ninth month the arrival of your baby is near. Do not try and worry about where you may be when your labor starts. All the distress that you will go threw will disappear at the sight of your new born baby.

Dealing with Changes of Third Trimester
During your third trimester you should have a calorie intake of 2400 calories. Eat small meals and snacks. Make sure to eat slow and chew your food well to aide with the digestion of it. To help with heartburn it is a good idea not to lie down right after eating. Consume less greasy foods and try and keep your head and shoulders raised. It is not advised to take water with meals. It is also advised that you do not consume alcohol, tobacco or coffee. The heartburn will go away so no need to worry about buying antacids. Ask your doctor how much fluid you should be taking in a day, stay away from sugar and caffeine filled drinks. Consume a prenatal vitamin rich in folic acid and other vitamins that you will need for your pregnancy. In the third trimester you shouldn't have any problems with cravings.

Back pain

Dealing with back pain during pregnancy is very common. You will probably experience back pain often during your third trimester. Make sure to take good posture to help with this, or get a massage that will help ease these aches.

Exercise

To reduce the swelling on your feet and ankles you can put your legs up and avoid the habit of crossing your legs. Make sure to wear comfortable clothing such as free flowing dresses. Do simple exercises such as walking and do easy house chores to keep your body moving. Make sure to alternate exercise with rest. You need to relax so that your baby can also relax. During your third trimester you should try to focus on exercises for joint mobility, flexibility and labor preparation. These moves will help strengthen your pelvic floor and keep your pelvis and hips mobile and will relieve discomfort as you prepare for labor. In the ninth month, yo need to try different sleeping positions because of the drastic tiredness you will be feeling.

Sleeping Stretch Pose. Lie on your back and interlock your fingers with both hands beneath your head then bend your knees keeping the soles of your feet on the floor then tilt your head in the opposite direction and repeat this process.

Butterfly Stretches. Try this stretch by stretching your legs out, bend the right knee and place your right foot on the left thigh as far as you can. Put your right hand on your right knee that is bent. Hold your toes of the right foot with your left hand. Gently move your right knee up towards your chest while you breath gently.

Cycling Horizontally. Lie down on your bed or yoga mat then air cycle with both your legs on an imaginary bike in the air.

Heartburn and Constipation

Your body increases its production of progesterone during pregnancy. This is the hormone that is responsible for relaxing your muscles including the esophagus. When these muscles relax they are unable to do their job in keeping foods down and acids. This can end up leading to heartburn. Try to keep away from spicy, acidic foods, and eat smaller meals throughout the day. To help relieve constipation you should increase your fiber intake. Also take more fluids. Contact your doctor if you have not had a bowel movement in three days.

Spider Veins

The increased circulation that you get when you are pregnant is to send blood to your growing baby. You could develop spider veins-red veins that develop on your skin. They will often appear early in your pregnancy, but they will get worse in the third trimester, do not worry they should fade after you give birth.

Varicose Veins

Besides suffering from spider veins you can also get varicose veins. These veins swell and are purple or blue in color. You can find relief by moving around during the day and propping up your feet. Also you can wear support hose. After you have given birth the varicose veins should improve.

Hemorrhoids

Due to the increase of weight during pregnancy it can result in hemorrhoids. Hemorrhoids are varicose veins that form around the anus. This can cause discomfort and itchiness as well as difficulty during a bowel movement. Sit in a warm tub for a few minutes to get relief from hemorrhoids. Ask your doctor if you can use stool softeners and hemorrhoid creams during your pregnancy.

Warm-up Contractions

Before you experience labor you may experience 'warm-up' contractions known as Braxton Hicks. These contractions tend to be weak and unpredictable as far as coming and going. But if these contractions are becoming regular and painful you may actually be going into labor and it will be time to contact the doctor.

Chapter 4 – Dealing with Relationships During Pregnancy

Even though this is a precious time in your life, pregnancy can shake things up in relationships. You may find yourself dealing with unsolicited advice, family members that are feeling neglected, strangers that want to feel your baby bump, reactions of co-workers to your pregnancy etc. These situations can certainly take a toll on you. You have to deal with certain issues when you become pregnant these are:

- ∞ When is a good time to announce your pregnancy.

- ∞ Depending on the relationships that you have with others will help determine when you will tell them about your pregnancy.

- ∞ Decide what family members and friends you will tell early on in pregnancy.

- ∞ When you should talk to your boss.

- ∞ Telling people that you are pregnant will explain why you are refusing an alcoholic beverage or for you to participate in an activity you should not do while pregnant etc.

- ∞ Finding the right moment to tell your partner. This is going to be the relationship that will change the most out of a pregnancy.

- ∞ Ask your partner what their feelings are on you being pregnant.

- ∞ Communicate to partner using touch.

- ∞ Allow your partner to bond with baby early on in pregnancy.

∞ You may want your growing baby inside you to grow in a nice clean environment, but you may be having trouble keeping up with things now that you are pregnant.

∞ Take your time when choosing a name for your baby. Make sure to chose a name that is not going to cause your baby pain in the future.

∞ Find out what your companies maternity leave rules are.

∞ Know your limits with work while pregnant.

∞ Knowing how to navigate your relationships will offer you great comfort during and after your pregnancy.

How to Get a Good Nights Sleep During Pregnancy

You are going to experience sleep disturbances as you go through your pregnancy when you need to deal with issues such as leg cramps, heartburn and nausea. You may also find yourself snoring due to the changes that are occurring in your body. To help improve the quality of your sleep during pregnancy you should:

∞ Cut down the caffeine intake you have.

∞ Try not to drink caffeine filled drinks in the afternoon or evening.

∞ You need to drink lots of fluids when you are pregnant.

∞ Drink more in the earlier part of the day and less in the evenings.

∞ Avoid eating spicy foods this can reduce your chances of getting heartburn

∞ Don't eat big heavy meals just before bed.

∞ Have a snack before bed then you will less likely be woken up with hunger pangs. This will also help to reduce nausea in the mornings.

∞ Take naps while pregnant, pregnancy can bring about shortness of breath and exhaustion.

∞ Help rest your mind and body by taking short naps, this way you will not be too tired to sleep at night.

∞ Give yourself a sleep schedule this will help your body get better prepared to go to sleep at bedtime.

∞ Create a nice soothing bedtime routine that will help get you ready for sleep.

∞ Make sure that you know what needs to be done for the next day so that you will not stay awake worrying.

∞ Make sure that your bedroom is not filled with clutter.

∞ Sleep on your left side for the sake of your baby. This will help your baby to get the nutrients and blood that it needs.

∞ If you are having trouble going to sleep then get up and do something relaxing and then go back to bed.

Chapter 5 –Dealing with Pregnancy Related Stress

It is certainly no joke when you have a growing life inside of you. Being pregnant brings with it its amount of stress for a new mother-to-be. Besides feeling anxiety about the health of your child, the birth process, and the changes in your life that will be brought on by a child being introduced into the mix can all be overwhelming, but you also have to deal with relationships and people around you. It is no wonder that you may feel stressed from time to time, but for the sake of your child you need to manage your stress.

One of the good steps towards managing your stress is to learn to say 'no' during your pregnancy. You will find that you are not going to be able to do as much as you used to before you became pregnant. Don't worry this is fine. Keep in mind that you are not a Superwoman and you have nothing to prove. Take this time to cut back on tasks and delegate work to others—loved ones, friends, and co-workers. If you have sick days or vacation, use these to have time to rejuvenate and rest your body.

Make sure that you are getting regular exercise. Exercise is beneficial to you whether you are pregnant or not. Doing regular exercise will help rejuvenate your mind and body. When you have a healthy body you will have less to worry about during your pregnancy.

Cut back on doing chores and remember that your baby comes first. Try to do deep breathing exercises in order to help calm yourself. Make sure to get enough sleep because you do no want to stress your baby out. Eating a well-balanced diet will help you to stay strong and healthy during your pregnancy. Try to avoid information overload during pregnancy, too much information about pregnancy can have you feeling stressed. Try to concentrate on being healthy instead of thinking about things that could go wrong. Join a support group if you are going through it alone. Sometimes it is nice to hear from others that everything will be okay.

Chapter 6 – Feeling Good About Your Body

When you are pregnant your body goes through various changes, it is easy for a new mother-to-be to feel overwhelmed. Your hormones will be working in overdrive as these changes occur in your body. You may feel that you are feeling really low especially where your body is concerned. Many women are sensitive to the changes that occur with their bodies during pregnancy. Instead of spending your time being focused on 'losing your looks', focus on feeling good about your body. You should:

∞ Stay active during your pregnancy.

∞ Do daily workout that will help keep you strong and healthy throughout your pregnancy

You may find that you have become less active due to feeling bloated or sick. However staying on the couch is not going to make you feel better. You need to exercise. Doing some yoga or going for a nice walk will help to lift your spirits and leave you feeling energized. You will build muscle tone and strength by exercising. This is going to help you to manage the weight and will help you to bounce back after your baby's birth.

Apply makeup to help you to feel that you are back in control of your life. Using makeup makes you feel pretty. If you are not one for using makeup then try out a new hairdo to give you a lift in spirits or get some new outfits for your pregnancy. Make sure to take good care of your skin you may find that it becomes dry during pregnancy. Use natural skin products on your belly to keep it moisturized. Treat yourself to a pregnancy massage. You will leave feeling good about your body.

You need to encourage positive thoughts during your pregnancy. The way that you view yourself in your mind is going to effect the way that you are feeling. Don't look at yourself in the mirror and see a fat lady, but instead look at yourself as a future mother-to-be and that you are carrying another growing healthy life inside of your belly. Look forward to meeting your baby. Keep in mind that the changes that you are going through during pregnancy are mostly temporary. Surround yourself with positive thoughts on this wonderful experience of becoming a new mother.

Preparing for Labor

You need to look into preparing for labor with the seriousness that it deserves. You do not want to be caught off guard when you go into labor. You need to be ready to do certain things when the time you have been waiting for is drawing nearer.

You need to first determine when to go to the hospital. Make sure that you are pre-registered at the hospital that you want to have your baby delivered in. Make choices on how you want the birth of your baby to be conducted. You should seek advice from your doctor when making these decisions. You need to fill out your plan for child form to guide the medics on how to go about the delivery to the best of your interests and that of your baby. Make sure that you have numbers for day and night contacts in case you should break your water in the middle of the night.

Make sure that you have your transportation arrangements, especially if you stay alone. Make sure that you have supplies that you will need for your newborn such as a car seat, nursing bras, baby bottles, diapers, cotton balls, baby's cap, crib sheet, mild soap. Don't buy too much stuff until you have your baby then you can purchase things to suit them.

Things to Pack for Hospital

Giving birth is something that takes time so you may want to make sure that you are going to be as comfortable as you can while in hospital. Pack clothes for you and your baby. Pack clothes for you that are comfortable and will not rub up on you and cause you discomfort. The clothes you choose should also make breast feeding easier. You may want to pack some flip flops as your feet may still be swollen. Your own personal towel. Your toiletries will add to your comfort. Bring your own pillow if you like. Pack camera or video camera, don't forget extra batteries. Bring your phone. Some crosswords or reading material to help time go by for you. Bring some snacks with you. Pacifiers for baby, nursing aids. It will be good to be prepared as you will be leaking. You may want to bring pads and extra underwear. It is best to pack all the things that you will need ahead of time. Packing a bag about a month before scheduled due date is a good idea as you could end up going into labor early. Make sure that you have all the documents you will need for your hospital stay.

Women have different experiences during labor some have more pain than others, no two pregnancies are the same. Make sure to follow what the doctors say so that you can have a safe delivery of your baby.

Conclusion

You are doing one of the most noble things in life in carrying a new life in your body. You are going to find that delivering a newborn is going to be one of the most fulfilling experiences in your life. I hope that you will find my tips and suggestions helpful to you through your nine month journey towards bringing new life into the world. Reading this book will help you to know basically what to expect through each trimester of your pregnancy, this will help ease the tension of your pregnancy. I wish to congratulate on becoming a new mother-to-be and also wish you a successful pregnancy!

If you found this book helpful I would really appreciate if you could leave a small review of it on Amazon. Thanks so much for your positive support is very appreciated!